CAT'S CLAW
(UNA DE GATO)

(Uncaria Tomentosa)

MIRACLE HERB FROM THE
RAIN FOREST OF PERU

© 1995 Copyright

Woodland Publishing Inc.
P.O. Box 160
Pleasant Grove, UT 84062

TABLE OF CONTENTS

INTRODUCTION

In a time when we are concerned with vital health issues that profoundly affect our families, Cat's Claw offers a potential powerhouse of therapeutic actions. Cat's Claw is currently drawing a great deal of attention in health-care circles, and within a relatively short time span, is experiencing dramatic worldwide demand. Because Cat's Claw has been accruing some impressive credentials in relation to its anti-tumor, anti-inflammatory and anti-viral capabilities, it has created a veritable frenzy of interest. It is currently widely used in Europe as a treatment for:

CANCER
AIDS
ARTHRITIS
SEVERAL OTHER DEGENERATIVE DISEASES

The emergence of Cat's Claw is a timely one. Because many individuals feel that the war on cancer is being lost, that new, potentially fatal viruses continue to evolve, and that the gross over-prescription of antibiotics has made us much more vulnerable to infection, taking herbal supplements like Cat's Claw is becoming more the rule than the exception.

All of us want to know how to:

- reduce our risk of cancer
- protect ourselves from toxins and pollutants
- boost our immune systems to fight off new viral strains and bacterial disease which no longer responds to antibiotics
- prevent premature aging and degenerative diseases such as arthritis, heart disease, and stroke

3

In addition, many of us have found that the notion of treating disease after the fact is much less desirable than the ability to protect and support our immune systems. A well nourished and healthy immune system can keep us from developing a whole host of diseases, including cancer. Any natural substance that fortifies immunity, works to scavenge free radicals as an effective antioxidant, and eases inflammation at the same time, will obviously draw a great deal of interest.

Cat's Claw has shown its ability to positively affect all of these concerns and has emerged from the scientific community as a botanical treasure even more valuable than Dr. Keplinger, who rediscovered the botanical in the Peruvian rain forest, may have originally presumed.

CAT'S CLAW

(Uncaria Tomentosa, Gmel. Rubiaceae)

COMMON NAMES: Una de Gato, Paraguayo, Garabato, Una de Gavilan, Hawk's Claw

NOTE: Uncaria guianensis is also known as Cat's Claw or Una de Gato in Spanish and is a related species. The genus of this species has sometimes been referred to as Ourouparia, which is no longer accepted as its name.

UNCARIA (Rubiaceae) HAS SEVERAL SPECIES INCLUDING:

uncaria attenuata	uncaria bernaysii	uncaria calophylla
uncaria elliptica	uncaria ferrea DC	uncaria gambir
uncaria guianensis	uncaria kawakamii	uncaria orientalis
uncaria pteropoda	uncaria rhyncophylla	

Obviously, many species of the genus Uncaria exist in nature. In fact there are over 30. Some Peruvian scientists believe that the tomentosa species, which is Cat's Claw, offers the most promise as a therapeutic agent. Uncaria guianensis is frequently confused with Uncaria tomentosa.

PLANT PARTS: edible inner bark of the vine, (Peruvian natives also use the leaves and roots of this plant, however the inner bark is the primary source of pharmacological activity).

ACTIVE COMPOUNDS: oxindole-alkaloids (pteropodine, isopteropodine, speciophyllline, uncarine, mitraphylline, isomitraphylline), N-oxide, rhynocophylline, N-oxide, carboline alkaloid, hirustine N-oxide triterpenes, polyphenols, phytosterols (stigmasterol and campsterol). The family of Rubiaceae, to which Cat's Claw belongs, is rich is triterpenoid saponins. Phytochemical studies of the root bark resulted in the isolation of the main alkaloid called isoteropodine. In addition, Peruvian and Italian researchers have discovered a whole host of phytochemicals including proanthocyanidin, which has already established itself as a powerful antioxidant.

PHARMACOLOGY: Uncaria tomentosa is an alkaloid-rich plant. Alkaloids exhibit a wide range of pharmacological and biological activities in the human body. They are nitrogen-containing organic compounds which can react with acids to form salts and are the basis of many medicines.

Cat's Claw possesses anti-inflammatory anti-edemic glycosides, which treat gastric ulcers, tumors and arthritis. Extracts of this plant have exhibited cytostatic and contraceptive actions as well.

Phytochemical studies have led to the isolation of a number of alkaloids found in Cat's Claw that have displayed the ability to enhance phagocytosis, thereby boosting the defense mechanisms of the immune system.

Laboratory studies at the University of Naples have isolated three new quinovic acid glycosides from the bark of Uncaria tomentosa.[1] Some of these new compounds displayed some antiviral activity and significant anti-inflammatory capabilities.[2] In addition, the oxindole alkaloids contained in the plant have demonstrated some antileukemic effects on cell walls,[3] suggesting that the herb may be of value as a treatment for leukemia.

NOTE: Laboratory tests have found that three varieties of the plant are related to climate, with the dark red type preferring a warm, and moist environment, the white-grey variety, cool and dry conditions and the yellow-brown type, somewhere in between.[4] No correlations could be found between the alkaloid content of the root bark and its color. It is true, however, that plants which have been harvested at different times can vary in their alkaloid content.[5]

CHARACTER: anti-inflammatory, anti-rheumatic, antioxidant, anti-viral, anti-tumor, anti-microbial, contraceptive, cytostatic activities, immune system enhancer

BODY SYSTEMS TARGETED: immune system, intestinal system, and cardiovascular system

TRADITIONAL TRIBAL HERBAL FORMS:

Peruvian natives have traditionally used Cat's Claw in a variety of interesting applications. They apply its leaves for headaches, use hot and cold decoctions or teas for infections such as influenza, and plants have been placed in antipyretic baths for fevers. Gargles are frequently used and poultices of the boiled crushed bark can be applied to affected areas. Traditional Peruvian tribal medicine has also vigorously rubbed decoctions or infusions of the raw bark on particular parts of the body, such as the limbs. Vines are frequently macerated with a hard wooden pestle or stems are allowed to stand in water for several hours. Snuffing or smoking dried leaves or bark occasionally occurs. Enemas, which have been used in some regions of tropical South American are relatively rare in the Amazon.

CURRENT FORMS OF CAT'S CLAW

- Dried, powdered form, usually available in gelatin capsules

- Compressed Tablets

- Decoction or Tea

- Liquid suspensions in the form of gels or extracts, which can be taken in soft gelatin capsule form

NOTE: Some experts believe that extracts of Uncaria tomentosa have not yet proven their potency and recommend taking reliable sources of the plant which use the inner bark of the vine. Because the alkaloid content of some plants can vary due to a number of different factors, only reputable sources of Cat's Claw should be purchased.

SAFETY: European studies have shown that Uncaria tomentosa has extremely low toxicity even when taken in large doses. It should not be taken, however by anyone who has had a transplant, or by pregnant or nursing women. Taking Cat's Claw may cause diarrhea or alter bowl consistency in some individuals.

CAT'S CLAW: A BRIEF HISTORY

WONDER HERB FROM THE AMAZONIAN RAIN FOREST OF PERU

Cat's Claw or Una de gato is a woody vine that comes to us from the exotic highlands and jungles of the Amazon rain forest. This dense, tropical rain forest spans an area of almost 2.3 million square miles and gives life to more plant and animal species than any other ecosystem on the planet. Estimates of different plant species which originate from this Amazon region place the figure somewhere between 35,000 and 80,000.

Even the most qualified botanist has a very limited knowledge of all the medicinal properties of Amazon rain forest flora. Finding an unusually bioactive plant is always exciting. Phytochemists have found a veritable storehouse of remarkable and diverse medicinal compounds in the Amazon.

The vegetal wealth of the region has provided modern man with a number of marvelous therapeutic herbs however, its potential has barely been tapped. It was by conserving and respecting the Peruvian folklore of this richly endowed region that a plant like Cat's Claw was rediscovered. Cat's Claw may be one of the Amazon's most impressive health-promoting gifts. Evidence strongly suggests that the alkaloid and phytochemical content of Cat's Claw may distinguish it as a wonder herb of the 21st century.

TRADITIONAL PERUVIAN TRIBAL MEDICINE

Both the bark and roots of this vine have been historically used by its indigenous native Peruvian tribes as an invaluable natural medicinal. Peruvian tribal folklore describes decoctions or teas made from the Uncaria tomentosa vine and their extraordinary ability to cure tumors, soothe arthritis, ease gastric upsets and boost the immune system.

Considered a sacred botanical by the local Indians, this vine grows wild in the highlands of the Peruvian Amazon in South America. Ashanica Indians have used both the bark and roots of the vine for generations on end to treat numerous health problems, targeting the immune and digestive systems in particular. Several Peruvian tribes have long valued Uncaria tea as an effective treatment for dysentery. Some have speculated that Una de Gato dates back to the time of the ancient Inca.

Obviously, medical science has not even begun to tap the incredible resource of therapeutic botanicals found in the rain forests. Tribal legend and practice must be sought out and recorded, or our understanding of these potentially life saving plants will be forever lost. Consider this quote:

"A large number of the trees forming these forests are still unknown to science, and yet the Indians, these practical botanists and zoologists, are well acquainted, not only with their external appearance, but also with their various properties..."[6]

UNCARIA TOMENTOSA: A PLANT WITH HOOKED CLAWS

The vine of what is technically the Uncaria tomentosa shrub, commonly grows in the foothills of the Amazon and along its river banks, taking a great deal of time to grow and mature. It isn't unusual for a Uncaria vine to take more than twenty years to reach full size, which can be over 100 feet in length. Uncaria species typically grow in jungle regions from the Amazonian Basin in the south, to the high jungle areas of Junin.

It's intriguing name, Una de Gato, which is Spanish for Cat's Claw, was generated by the thorns which cover the vine and look very much like the claws of a cat. These stout, hooked spines enable the vine to wind itself up among the Peruvian trees seeking after more light amidst the deep shade of the canopied forest.

The vine produces a yellowish or white flower which blooms in pairs on opposite sides of the stem. These are small dense, fragrant heads which are easily pollinated. The curled peduncles of the vine will eventually harden into hooks instead of remaining green. While the leaves of the vine are attractive and glossy, the sharp, curved, claw-like spines effectively keep intruders away. Men have literally been caught up by the vine's formidable hooks and have found themselves suspended in mid-air.[7]

Current harvesting of the Uncaria Tomentosa vine involves only the bark. The roots of the vine are carefully protected in order to preserve the plant and further its propagation. It is crucial to keep in mind that the many precious plant species of the rain forests of the world must be conserved and protected.

THE KEPLINGER CONNECTION TO CAT'S CLAW

In 1974, Cat's Claw was discovered anew by Klaus Keplinger. Through personal conversations with the Ashanica Indians, he learned that medical doctors had shown considerable interest in the plant. In July of 1989 and 1990, two patents were issued to Keplinger for isolating six alkaloid compounds from the root of the plant.[8] The patents stipulate that these alkaloids are "suitable for the unspecific stimulation of the immune system."[9]

Clinical studies involving Cat's Claw began in the 1970's and have been ongoing ever since. Research which has emerged from facilities in Germany, Austria, Italy, Hungary, England and Peru suggest that Cat's Claw may be a viable treatment for several significant diseases and disorders which are discussed in a later section.

Recently, a medical doctor in Austria developed a pharmaceutical from an extract of Cat's Claw and caused a great deal of interest in the herb. Apparently, he has successfully used extracts of Cat's Claw to treat people suffering from AIDS and cancer. This physician was well acquainted with the therapeutic history of this vine and its traditional usage by the Ashanika Indians.

DR. BRENT DAVIS AND CURRENT EVALUATIONS OF CAT'S CLAW

Dr. Brent Davis, who had become fascinated with Cat's Claw long before it emerged as a natural health supplement refers to Uncaria tomentosa as "the opener of the way" referring to its unique ability to detoxify the intestinal tract and to treat a variety of stomach and bowel disorders.[10]

In 1988, an international congress was held in Lima, Peru to share information on traditional Peruvian therapies. Several physicians lauded Cat's Claw and one specifically cited his use of the herb to successfully treat 14 types of confirmed cases of cancer in 700 patients between 1984 and 1988.[11]

In November of the same year, articles dealing with the medicinal actions of Uncaria Tomentosa or Cat's Claw appeared in El Commercio a major newspaper published in Lima, Peru. The article addressed the medicinal potential of Krallendon, an extract of the plant, which had been tested by Dr. Keplinger at Immodel in Austria. The results which

Dr. Keplinger had seen with this extract in working with allergies, genital herpes, herpes zoster, neurobronchitis, cancer and even AIDS was provocative, to say the least. In her book, *Witch Doctor's Apprentice, Hunting for Medicinal Plants in the Amazonian,* 3rd Edition, Nicole Maxwell discloses that Sidney McDaniel has submitted samples of Cat's Claw to the NIH cancer screen.[12]

In 1992, Italian researchers from the University of Milan found that along with its many other attributes, Cat's Claw acts as a powerful antioxidant as well. Uncaria is currently exported by the tons to Europe for the treatment of various kinds of cancer. In Peru, anyone can readily obtain Cat's Claw at local pharmacies.

PERUVIAN HARVESTING LAWS AND UNCARIA TOMENTOSA

The demand for Cat's Claw has dramatically escalated over the last several years. Countries all over the world are ordering the herb in extremely large quantities, so much so that estimates predict that both Uncaria species would become extinct within the next five years.[13] Vines seldom constitute more than 10% of stems found in natural forests.[14]

The Peruvian government has taken certain important steps to ensure that supplies of Uncaria tomentosa will not become exhausted due to imprudent harvesting. Unfortunately, other South American countries have permitted the tragic destruction of their precious rain forests and other ecosystems. Peruvian legislation has made harvesting the root of both Uncaria tomentosa and Uncaria guianensis illegal.

This ruling is not problematic for medical botanists because the bark contains all the therapeutic attributes of the herb. The edible bark of both species grows back and continually replenishes itself. On the other hand, extricating or cutting the root causes the vine to perish.

The pharmacopoeial wealth of the Amazonian region holds the medical miracle drugs and herbals of the future. It is literally impossible to begin to decipher and chemically analyze all of the indigenous native flora, therefore, it is better to concentrate first on those species which have been found by the local peoples to have medicinal effects. This is precisely what occurred with Uncaria tomentosa.

CLINICAL RESEARCH ON CAT'S CLAW HAS BEEN CONDUCTED AT:

- University of Innsbruck, Austria

- University of Munich, Germany

- The Huntington Research Center, England

- The Central Research Institute of Chemistry, Hungary

- The University of Milan, Italy

- The University of Naples, Italy

- Several Peruvian Research Facilities

FUNCTIONS

Cat's Claw has traditionally been used to treat arthritis, gastritis, tumors, dysentery and female hormonal imbalances. Today, the plant has demonstrated the ability to treat **viral infections, minimize inflammation, and provide therapeutic action for a variety of stomach and bowel disorders including: arthritis, Crohn's Disease, ulcers, gastritis, parasites, diverticulitis, hemorrhoids, several types of cancer, irritable bowel syndrome, herpes, allergies, lupus, diabetes, PMS, yeast infections, hypoglycemia, prostatitis, bursitis, and rheumatism.**

Currently, European studies are looking to isolates of Cat's Claw for their ability to treat **AIDS and cancer.** The following section addresses specific conditions in more detail as they relate to Cat's Claw. Philip N. Steinberg, a Certified Nutritional consultant has stated:

"Uncaria tomentosa has so many therapeutic applications that it seems to far surpass such well known herbs as Pau d'arco, echinacea, goldenseal, astragalus, Artemesia annua, Siberian and Panax ginseng, as well as maitake, shiitake and reishi mushrooms and other natural products including, grapefruit seed extract, caprylic and lauric acids and shark cartilage."[15]

Steinberg had the opportunity to speak with Dr. Satya Ambrose, co-founder of the Oregon College of Oriental Medicine concerning Cat's Claw. Within months of using it in capsule form, she has observed some very impressive results in treating **Crohn's disease, ulcers, fibromyalgia and asthma.**[16]

Phillip Steinberg has experimented with the herb since September of 1993. He relates:

"I, along with my wife, children, some friends and associates have been experimenting with Cat's Claw tea as well as capsules. We have found both to be effective in knocking out the flu, clearing up sinus, ear and upper respiratory infections, canker sores, one infection associated with TMJ, eliminating lower back pain associated with arthritis and eliminating the tired sore muscles associated with heavy physical work and exercise. I was even able to clear up a case of athlete's foot by putting the powdered herb between the infected toes, and my daughter's conjunctivitis by putting drops of the tea in her eyes several times over the course of two days. Even more amazing is that all the above were accomplished within 48 hours after beginning use of the herb."[17]

PRIMARY APPLICATIONS OF CAT'S CLAW INCLUDE:

- Allergies
- Arthritis
- Bursitis
- Cancer
- Candida (Yeast Infections)
- Chemotherapy
- Chronic Fatigue Syndrome
- Cirrhosis
- Crohn's Disease
- Edema
- Female Hormonal Imbalances
- Fibromyalgia
- Hemorrhoids
- Hormonal Imbalances
- Inflammation
- Intestinal Disorders
- Immune System
- Lupus
- Parasites
- PMS
- Radiation Treatments or Exposure
- Toxic Poisoning
- Ulcers
- Viral Infections (Influenza, Respiratory Infections)

In addition, the herb has also bee used for Athlete's Foot, Ear infections, diverticulitis, diabetes, hypoglycemia conjunctivitis, back pain, TMJ syndrome, prostatitis, bursitis, fibromyalgia, canker sores, sinus infections and asthma.

SPECIFIC DISORDERS TARGETED BY CAT'S CLAW

GASTROINTESTINAL DISORDERS AND THE ACTION OF CAT'S CLAW

When Dr. Brent Davis referred to Cat's Claw as "the opener of the way" he was alluding to the plants impressive ability to clear and cleanse the entire intestinal tract. Today, more than ever, the health status of the colon is considered a barometer for the rest of the body. In other words, a poorly functioning colon can be related to the development of a number of degenerative diseases including cancer. Traditionally, established medical practices have virtually ignored the colon's role in promoting disease. Today, ever emerging research is supporting the notion that keeping the colon clean and well functioning is vital to preventing disease and maintaining health.

"Breast Disease has been linked to the western diet and bowel dysfunction. There is an association between cellular abnormalities in breast fluid and the frequency of bowel movements.[18] This association is probably due to the bacterial flora in the large intestine transforming colon contents into a variety of toxic metabolites, including carcinogens and mutagens."[19]

Dr. Davis strongly advocated the use of Cat's Claw to treat various bowel diseases, especially those that harbored infection. He strongly believes that Uncaria tomentosa can successfully treat intestinal disease that has been so severe, it has not responded to other therapeutic substances. In addition, the role of friendly bacteria in the bowel cannot be overemphasized. Most bowel diseases are associated with a disruption in this beneficial flora. When intestinal flora is out of balance, the immune system can become compromised as well. In a 1992 report, Dr. Davis summarized,

"Derangement of human intestinal microflora is a common problem with the potential of fundamentally disrupting numerous metabolic pathways, producing diverse, unhealthy symptomatologies. Cat's Claw is a world class herb which has the power to arrest and reverse deep seated pathology, allowing a more rapid return to health."[20]

BOWEL DISORDERS WHICH REFLECT A TOXIC COLON INCLUDE:

- **Colitis**
- **Colon Cancer**
- **Constipation**
- **Crohn's Disease**
- **Diarrhea and Gas**
- **Diverticulitis**
- **Irritable Bowel Syndrome**

Dr. Davis believes that Cat's Claw can effectively detoxify the entire intestinal tract and contribute to the replenishment of friendly bacteria.

THE ANTI-INFLAMMATORY PROPERTIES OF CAT'S CLAW

For generations, Peruvians have trusted in the anti-inflammatory attributes of Cat's Claw. It has traditionally been used for any type of rheumatism or arthritic joint condition.

Clinical studies on the plant metabolites of Cat's Claw have discovered that it does indeed inhibit the inflammatory response. The plant sterols found in Cat's Claw exhibited the ability to reduce artificially induced swelling in the paws of rats. Using a test group and a control group, paw swelling was measured at hourly intervals for 5 hours. The inhibitory effects of plant sterols from Cat's Claw were calculated.

Interestingly, when these scientists separated these compounds and tested them separately, their anti-inflammatory properties became either completely inactive or inhibited. Consequently, the research team concluded that the strong anti-inflammatory activity of Cat's Claw extracts may be due to the presence of all the compounds together. They hypothesized that some of the compounds have an intrinsic anti-inflammatory effect, while other compounds may act synergistically to enhance their biological activity.[21]

This only serves to confirm what herbalists have strongly advocated for generations; that plants are designed to be used in their whole form to be biochemically effective. One of the reasons that pharmaceutical synthetic versions of herbal medications have so many bad side effects is that they have been chemically extricated and isolated. In so doing, the very crucial role of other compounds vital to the function of the plant are eliminated. Natural botanical remedies have been designed by Mother Nature to work synergistically.

Natural anti-inflammatories are so important for treating diseases such as arthritis and allergies because they have far less side effects than prescription NSAID'S, which are currently used by thousands of afflicted individuals. Back pain, joint pain, inflammation caused by histamine release and a whole host of other infirmities have resulted in the purchase of millions of dollars of anti-inflammatory drugs such as ibuprofen and naprosyn.

CAT'S CLAW: A POWERFUL IMMUNE SYSTEM BOOSTER

Devastating disease like AIDS and flesh-eating viruses have received considerable press coverage over the last several years. While most of us may not feel immediately threatened by these viruses, we may not be as immunologically strong as we could be. Most of us tumble from doctor to doctor, battling a neverending list of ailments including: colds, flu, sore throats, earaches, athlete's foot, yeast infections, chronic fatigue syndrome, herpes, colitis ect. ect. ect.. Heart disease, cancer, arthritis, and diabetes are responsible for thousands of deaths annually. Our country, as a whole, receives a poor bill of health.

Our immune systems are our built-in defense departments and must be kept in optimal working condition. Infectious microorganisms and carcinogens constantly surround us. Our immune systems are designed to fight off or neutralize the potential health threats of bacteria, viruses, fungi, and cancer cells. A healthy immune system has extraordinary abilities to ward off disease or minimize its stay. Fortifying our defenses with certain herbs, vitamins and antioxidants can go a long way to promote wellness.

Traditionally, the Uncaria tomentosa plant has been used in South American to treat disorders which are usually connected in one way or the other with the immune system. Through liquid chromatography, Gerhard Laus and Dietmar Keplinger isolated and identified six oxindole alkaloids from the plant.[22]

The two patents that were issued to Keplinger deal with its immuno-stimulatory properties. According to the patent, Isopteropodin is the most immunologically active of the alkaloids.

Clinical studies conducted by Keplinger found that four of the alkaloids found in Cat's Claw exhibit significant activity on phagocytosis. Phagocytosis is the process in which certain white blood cells called macrophages attack and literally digest infectious organisms and foreign invaders.

A clinical study conducted at the University of Naples confirmed the fact that Cat's Claw alkaloids "display a pronounced enhancement of phagocytosis."[23] Bark was collected and identified and a voucher sample was deposited at the Herbarium of the University. The three alkaloids which were studied were new quinovic acid alkaloids. These compounds were investigated through chemical analysis.

VIRAL INFECTIONS

As a natural anti-viral and immune system booster, Philip Steinberg believes that Cat's Claw may be more effective than both Echinacea and Pau d'arco. Krallendon, an extract of Uncaria tomentosa is the bioactive component of the plant which Dr. Keplinger used to successfully treat genital herpes, herpes zoster and AIDS, which are all viral diseases.

Various biological activities have been attributed to the triterpenoid saponins found in Cat's Claw. Glycoside glycyrrhizin and glycyrrhetinic acid have exhibited the ability to inhibit the multiplication of some DNA viruses.[24] In addition all nine compounds tested showed an inhibitory effect against the vesicular stomatitis virus when used in certain concentrations. In other words, Cat's Claw can fight certain kinds of infection.

These new quinovic acid glycosides have been isolated from Uncaria tomentosa. In addition during the course of another chemical search for biologically active metabolites from the plant, three new triterpenes were discovered.[25]

AIDS

Krallendon, which is the commercialized name for one of the constituents of Uncaria tomentosa has been used to treat AIDS patients either as an isolated treatment or in conjunction with AZT. This combination apparently helps to inhibit the reproduction of the HIV virus in the blood while it simultaneously activates the immune system. This same effect was seen on cancerous cells.[26] Studies have suggested that when this alkaloid was used, side effects typically associated with AZT therapy and with traditional cancer treatments were reduced as well.[27]

Dr. Keplinger has used Krallendon to treat seven AIDS patients who were in different stages of the disease. According to the article published in El Commercio in Lima, Peru, he helped all but two of them. The article states that the other five patients experienced such a dramatic improvement that symptoms of the disease disappeared.[28]

For the past six years, Dr. Keplinger has used Krallendon to treat his AIDS patients. According to Immodal, none of their symptoms have continued to escalate. In other words, they are holding their own.

"The cases that displayed the first symptoms of the disease showed an improvement in blood analysis and a disappearance of clinical symptoms within the first year; and in Immodal's own words, `a situation that continues to this day.'"[29]

CAT'S CLAW AND CANCER

European health practitioners are currently testing and using Cat's Claw as a potential treatment for various cancers. The unprecedented amount of Cat's Claw which is shipped to several European countries may be related to its anti-carcinogenic reputation.

One Peruvian doctor has reported to his colleagues that he had successfully used Uncaria tomentosa and other herbs in treating 14 types of accurately diagnosed cancer in 700 patients between 1984 and 1988.[30]

Cat's Claw may work to lower the risk of cancer in two ways. It has the ability to act as an antioxidant and may scavenge for carcinogenic substances which can cause the formation of cancerous cells. In addition, scientific studies have shown that it can specifically target cellular mutations such as leukemic cells and inhibit their development.

During the course of Austrian research on Cat's Claw, its oxindole alkaloids were tested for their antileukemic effects on cells which may suggest that these compounds have value as treatments for leukemia. Colormetric testing was only one of the ways the compounds were tested and showed that all of the oxindole alkaloids, with the exception of one, inhibited the growth of certain leukemic cells.[31] Interestingly, while leukemic cell activity was inhibited, normal bone marrow cells were not affected. This ability of the compound to differentiate between leukemic cells and normal stem cells strongly suggests that Uncaria tomentosa or Cat's Claw should be considered as a viable treatment for people with acute leukemia.[32] For anyone undergoing cancer treatment, Cat's Claw can act as a support to the entire physiological system.

CAT'S CLAW SUPPORTS THE BODY DURING CHEMOTHERAPY AND RADIATION TREATMENTS, WORKING AS AN ANTIOXIDANT IN HELPING TO REMOVE TOXIC METABOLITES AND IN PROVIDING SUPPORT TO AN ALREADY WEAKENED IMMUNE SYSTEM.

THE ANTIOXIDANT ACTION OF CAT'S CLAW

It's a scientific fact that most of us will not live out our potential maximum life spans. Unfortunately, because of the damage that free radicals cause within our cellular structures, many of us will die prematurely from one of a wide variety of degenerative diseases. Free radicals are nothing more than unstable molecular structures which pose a threat to healthy organic tissue by randomly assaulting cellular structures.

The very act of breathing oxygen creates reactive chemical structures known as free radicals. To make matters worse, because our generation is exposed to a number of potentially harmful environmental pollutants, free radical formation can reach critical levels.

Several studies have concluded that Uncaria isolates have several beneficial constituents which act as free radical scavengers. The polyphenols, triterpines and plant steroids contribute to the antioxidant capabilities of Cat's Claw. Isolates of the plant have the ability to protect the cells from mutating, which is what occurs when tumors develop.

This anti-mutagenic activity was observed by Italian researchers in 1992, at the University of Milan. Smoking is one of the worst sources of oxidative stress caused by the release of millions of free radicals. These Italian researchers studied the effects of an aqueous alcoholic infusion of Uncaria tomentosa on people who smoke.

"Urine samples of healthy donors: half smokers, the other half non-smokers were collected before, during and after treatment. While the non-smoker's urine did not show any mutagenic activity, the smoker's urine exhibited decreased mutagenic potential by the end of the treatment, persisting for eight days after the end of treatment. The Italian team concluded, `This plant shows anti-mutagenic activity in-vivo in smokers, confirming its high antioxidant potential.'"[33]

To really appreciate the significance of this study one must be aware of the very real perils of cigarette smoke. Even passive smokers who are only exposed to second hand smoke experience a surge of oxidants on a cellular level.

"Smokers, a group at high risk from heart disease and cancer, inhale large amounts of potentially injurious free radicals derived from tobacco...The elevation in conjugated dienes in plasma indicates that smokers incur abnormal oxidative stress...It is possible that a prolonged increase in antioxidant intake could ameliorate free radical-mediated damage in smokers and thereby decrease the risk of developing diseases such as coronary heart disease and cancer."[34]

In addition to cigarette smoke, Cat's Claw can also

help protect cells from a number of potentially harmful environmental substances including:

- herbicides
- pesticides
- smog
- car exhaust
- certain prescription and over-the-counter drugs
- diagnostic and therapeutic x-rays
- ultra-violet light
- gamma radiation
- rancid foods
- certain fats
- alcohol
- stress
- poor diets, (high fat, high protein)

CAT'S CLAW: A SOURCE OF PROANTHOCYANIDIN (PYCNOGENOL)

The wealth of phytochemicals inherent to the Uncaria tomatosa plant include proanthocyanidins, which have strongly established themselves as potent antioxidants. Four dimeric procyanidins have been shown to constitute a portio of the plant extract.[35]

Proanthocyanidins are found in Pycnogenol, and are commonly extracted from grape seeds or pine bark. Proanthocyanidins have accrued an impressive list of antioxidant bioactivity and promise to attract a great deal more attention in the near future.

Because proanthocyanidins scavenge free radicals so effectively, they have shown some remarkable curative effects. Extensive research has demonstrated that proanthocyanidins are such potent antioxidants that they can find and neutralize free radicals with great rapidity, allowing cells to regenerate rather than deteriorate. They have extremely high bioavailability. Specific actions associated with proanthocyanidins include:

- capillary protection which helps prevent varicose veins, phlebitis and excess bruising
- significant anti-inflammatory action in cases of joint pain and injuries
- anti-edemic, in that it helps control swelling and reduce water retention
- antihistamine, in that it decreases the production of histamine commonly seen in allergic reactions
- reduces the risk of diabetic complications such as retinopathy

It's interesting to note that proanthocyanidins target many of the same disorders that Cat's Claw is also used for. The addition of important alkaloids to the proantho-cyanidins in Cat's Claw make it an herbal panacea for cellular protection against a number of diseases and environmental toxins.

CARDIOVASCULAR DISEASE AND CAT'S CLAW

Estimates predict that 50% or more of our population will suffer from heart disease. The inordinate amount of attention given to changing diet and lifestyle has improved cardiovascular health to some degree, however, in general, it has not significantly reduced the incidence of cardiovascular disease. Several factors contribute to heart disease including our exposure to oxidants.

Cat's Claw works to scavenge for free radicals, which frequently damage arterial walls, resulting in high blood pressure, heart disease and death from either heart attack or stroke. While cholesterol levels and the type of dietary fat we consume significantly contribute to cardiovascular disease, the tendency of blood to coagulate is also crucial. Cat's Claw discourages blood from clotting.

The rynchophylline found in Cat's Claw has proven itself to be an inhibitor of platelet formation and thrombosis. In lay terms, this means that it inhibits the formation of blood clots.[36] What this suggests is that the alkaloid compounds in Cat's Claw may reduce the risk of stroke and heart attack. Cat's Claw enhances the circulation of blood and lessens the formation of arterial plaque deposits.

Many people are currently using aspirin therapy as a way to keep the blood thinned and reduce the risk of heart attack or stroke. Herbal blood thinners, such as Cat's Claw should be investigated as an another preventative therapy.

SUMMARY

Cat's Claw is nothing less than a wonder herb. Scientific studies have proven its medicinal worth. It should be used not only to treat a variety of modern-day diseases but as a preventative supplement as well. What Peruvian Indians have known for generations should be shared with the rest of the world in our struggle to conquer disease and maintain health.

ENDNOTES

[1]Riccardo Cerri, "New Quinovic Acid Glycosides from Uncaria tomentosa," *Journal of Natural Medicine,* Vol. 51, No. 2, Mar-Apr, 1988 257-261.

[2]Rita Aquino, Vincenzo De Feo, Francesco De Simone, Cosimo Pizza and Giuseppe Cirino, "Plant Metabolites, New Compounds and Anti-inflammatory Activity of Uncaria tomentosa," *Journal of Natural Products,* Vol. 54, No. 2, Mar-Apr, 1991, 453-459.

[3]H. Stuppner, S. Strum, G. Geisen, U. Zillian, and G. Konwalinka, "A Differential Sensitivity of Oxindole Alkaloids to Normal and Leukemic Cell Lines," *Planta Medica* 59, Supplement Issue, 1993, A583.

[4]Gerard Laus and Dietmar Keplinger, "Separation of Stereoisomeric Oxindole Alkaloids from Uncaria tomentosa by High Performance Liquid Chromatography," A, 662, 1994, 243-249.

[5]Ibid.

[6]Richard Evans Schultes. *Where Gods Reign, Plants and People of the Columbian Amazon.* (Oracle, Arizona: Synergetic Press, 1988), 28.

[7]Richard Spruce, Ph.D. *Notes of a Botanist on the Amazon and Andes.* (London: Macmillan and Co. 1908), 30.

[8]Philip N. Steinberg, "Uncaria tomentosa (Cat's Claw) A Wondrous Herb from the Peruvian Rainforest," *Townsend Letter,* #130, May, 1994, 2.

[9]Ibid.

[10]Philip A. Steinberg, "Uncaria tomentosa (Cat's Claw) Wonder Herb from the Amazon," *New Editions Health World,* February, 1995, 41.

[11]Ibid., 43.

[12]James Alan Duke and Rodolfo Vasquez. *Amazonian Ethnobotanical Dictionary.* (Boca Raton: CRC Press, 1994), 172.

[13]Steinberg, *New Editions,* 45.

[14]Francis E. Putz and Harold A. Mooney. *The Biology of Vines.* (Cambridge: Cambridge University Press, 1991), 330.

[15]Steinberg, *New Editions,* 43.

[16]Ibid.

[17]Ibid., 45.

[18]Michael Murray, N.D. and Joseph Pizzorno, N.D. *Encyclopedia of Natural Healing*. (Rocklin, California: Prima Publishing, 1991), 303. See also, N. L. Petrakis and E. B. King, "Cytological Abnormalities is Nipple Aspirates of Breast Fluid from Women with Severe Constipation," *Lancet* 1981, ii, 1203-05.

[19]Ibid., 303.

[20]"The Cat's Claw," *The Energy Times*, May-June, 1995, 12.

[21]Aquino, 453.

[22]Laus and Keplinger, 245.

[23]Cerri, 257.

[24]R. Aquino, F. De Simone and C. Pizza, "Plant Metabolites. Structure and In Vitro Antiviral Activity of Quinovic Acid Glycosides from Uncaria tomentosa and Guettarda platypoda," *Journal of Natural Products*, Vol. 52, No. 4. Jul-Aug, 1989, 679-685.

[25]R. Aquino, F. De Simone, F.F. Vincieri and C. Pizza, "New Polyhydroxylated Treiterpenes from Uncaria tomentosa," *Journal of Natural Products*, Vol. 53, No. 3, May-June, 1990, 559-564.

[26]Steinberg, *New Editions*, 44.

[27]Pat. Huemoller, "Cat's Claw," *Wellness Advocate*, Vol. 5 Issue 1, February, 1995.

[28]Steinberg, *New Editions*, 44.

[29]Ibid.

[30]Steinberg, *New Editions*, 43.

[31]Stuppner, 583.

[32]Ibid.

[33]"The Cat's Claw," 12.

[34]G.G. Duthie, "Antioxidant Status of Smokers and Non-Smokers," *Annal New York Academy of Sciences*, 1987, 435-438.

[35]S.M. de Matta, F.D. Monache, F. Ferrari and G.B. Bettolo, "Alkaloids and Procyanidins of an Uncaria Species from Eastern Peru," *Farmaco-Sci*, July, 1976, 31(7) 527-35.

[36]Steinberg, *New Editions*, 44.

INDEX